Table of Contents

1. A Consumer's Guide To The Nation's Drinking Water

The United States enjoys one of the best supplies of drinking water in the world. Nevertheless, many of us who once gave little or no thought to the water that comes from our taps are now asking the question: "Is my water safe to drink?" While tap water that meets federal and state standards is generally safe to drink, threats to drinking water are increasing. Short-term disease outbreaks and water restrictions during droughts have demonstrated that we can no longer take our drinking water for granted.

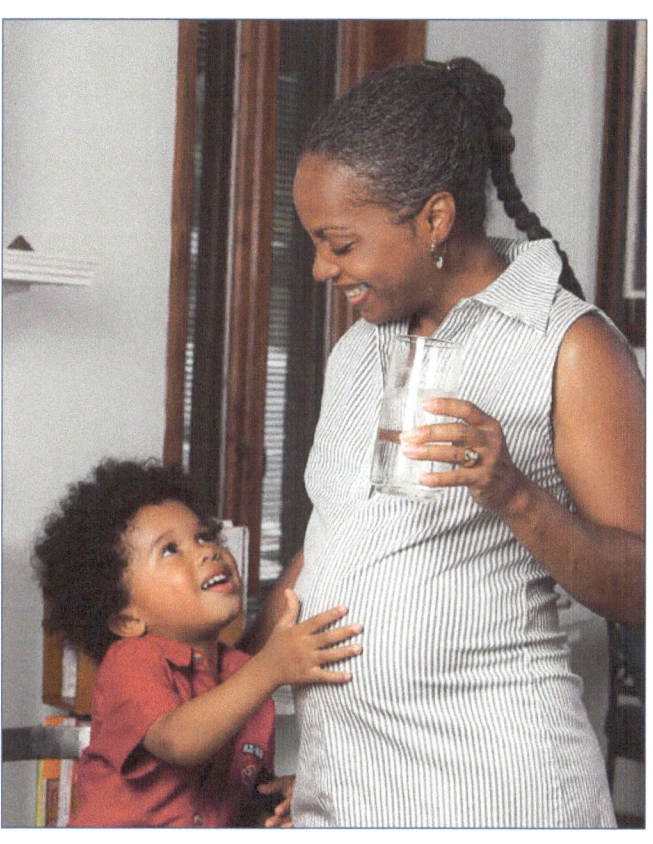

Consumers have many questions about their drinking water. How safe is my drinking water? What is being done to improve security of public water systems? Where does my drinking water come from, and how is it treated? Do private **wells** receive the same protection as public water systems? What can I do to help protect my drinking water?

This booklet provides the answers to these and other frequently asked questions.

This booklet also directs you to more detailed sources of information. Often, you will be directed to a page on the EPA website. Additionally, the Safe Drinking Water Hotline is available to answer your questions. Please also see Appendix C for more resources. Refer to the Glossary (Appendix D) for definitions of words in bold font.

What you need to know to protect your family

Sensitive Subpopulations

Some people may be more vulnerable to contaminants in drinking water than the general population. People undergoing chemotherapy or living with HIV/AIDS, transplant patients, children and infants, the frail elderly, and pregnant women and their fetuses can be particularly at risk for infections.

If you have special health care needs, consider taking additional precautions with your drinking water, and seek advice from your health care provider. For more information, see www.epa.gov/safewater/healthcare/special.html.

You will find information on bottled water and home water treatment units on page 16 of this booklet. You may also contact NSF International, Underwriter's Laboratory, or the Water Quality Association. Contact information is located in Appendix C.

2. How Safe Is My Drinking Water?

What Law Keeps My Drinking Water Safe?

Congress passed the Safe Drinking Water Act (SDWA) in 1974 to protect public health by regulating the nation's public drinking water supply and protecting sources of drinking water. SDWA is administered by the U.S. Environmental Protection Agency (EPA) and its state partners.

Highlights of the Safe Drinking Water Act

- Authorizes EPA to set enforceable health standards for contaminants in drinking water

- Requires public notification of water systems violations and annual reports (Consumer Confidence Reports) to customers on contaminants found in their drinking water - www.epa.gov/safewater/ccr

- Establishes a federal-state partnership for regulation enforcement

- Includes provisions specifically designed to protect underground sources of drinking water - www.epa.gov/safewater/uic

- Requires disinfection of surface water supplies, except those with pristine, protected sources

- Establishes a multi-billion-dollar state revolving loan fund for water system upgrades - www.epa.gov/safewater/dwsrf

- Requires an assessment of the vulnerability of all drinking water sources to contamination - www.epa.gov/safewater/protect

— Drinking Water: Past, Present, and Future
EPA-816-F-00-002

What Is A Public Water System?

The Safe Drinking Water Act (SDWA) defines a **public water system (PWS)** as one that serves piped water to at least 25 persons or 15 service connections for at least 60 days each year. There are approximately 161,000 public water systems in the United States.[1] Such systems may be publicly or privately owned. **Community water systems (CWSs)** are public water systems that serve people year-round in their homes. Most people in the U.S. (268 million) get their water from a community water system. EPA also regulates other kinds of public water systems,

Public Water Systems

Community Water System (54,000 systems)— A public water system that serves the same people year-round. Most residences are served by Community Water Systems.

Non-Community Water System (approximately 108,000 systems)—A public water system that does not serve the same people year-round. There are two types of non-community systems:

- Non-Transient Non-Community Water System (almost 19,000 systems)—A non-community water system that serves the same people more than six months of the year, but not year-round. For example, a school with its own water supply is considered a non-transient system.

- Transient Non-Community Water System (more than 89,000 systems)—A non-community water system that serves the public but not the same individuals for more than six months. For example, a rest area or a campground may be considered a transient system.

such as those at schools, campgrounds, factories, and restaurants. Private water supplies, such as household wells that serve one or a few homes, are not regulated by EPA. For information on household wells, see "How Safe Is The Drinking Water In My Household Well?" on page 18 of this booklet.

Will Water Systems Have Adequate Funding In The Future?

Nationwide, drinking water systems have spent hundreds of billions of dollars to build drinking water treatment and **distribution systems**. From 1995 to 2000, more than $50 billion was spent on capital investments to fund water quality improvements.[2]

With the aging of the nation's infrastructure, the clean water and drinking water industries face a significant challenge to sustain and advance their achievements in protecting public health. EPA's *Clean Water & Drinking Water Infrastructure Gap Analysis*[3] has found that if present levels of spending do not increase, there will be a significant funding gap by the year 2019.

Where Can I Find Information About My Local Water System?

Since 1999, water suppliers have been required to provide annual Consumer Confidence Reports to their customers. These reports are due by July 1 each year, and contain information on contaminants found in the drinking water, possible health effects, and the water's source. Some Consumer Confidence Reports are available at *www.epa.gov/safewater/dwinfo.htm.*

Water suppliers must promptly inform you if your water has become contaminated by something that can cause immediate illness. Water suppliers have 24 hours to inform their customers of **violations** of EPA standards "that have the potential to have serious adverse effects on human health as a result of short-term exposure." If such a violation occurs, the water system will announce it through the media, and must provide information about the potential adverse effects on human health, steps the system is taking to correct the violation, and the need to use alternative water supplies (such as boiled or bottled water) until the problem is corrected.

3

Systems will inform customers about violations of less immediate concern in the first water bill sent after the violation, in a Consumer Confidence Report, or by mail within a year. In 1998, states began compiling information on individual systems, so you can evaluate the overall quality of drinking water in your state. Additionally, EPA must compile and summarize the state reports into an annual report on the condition of the nation's drinking water. To view the most recent annual report, see *www.epa.gov/safewater/annual.*

How Often Is My Water Supply Tested?

EPA has established pollutant-specific minimum testing schedules for public water systems. To find out how frequently your drinking water is tested, contact your water system or the agency in your state in charge of drinking water.

If a problem is detected, immediate retesting requirements go into effect along with strict instructions about how the system informs the public. Until the system can reliably demonstrate that it is free of problems, the retesting is continued.

In 2001, one out of every four community water systems did not conduct testing or report the results for all of the monitoring required to verify the safety of their drinking water.[4] Although failure to monitor does not necessarily suggest safety problems, conducting the required reporting is crucial to ensure that problems will be detected. Consumers can help make sure certain monitoring and reporting requirements are met by first contacting their state drinking water agency to determine if their water supplier is in compliance. If the water system is not meeting the requirements, consumers can work with local and state officials and the water supplier to make sure the required monitoring and reporting occurs.

A network of government agencies monitor tap water suppliers and enforce drinking water standards to ensure the safety of public water supplies. These agencies include EPA, state departments of health and environment, and local public health departments.

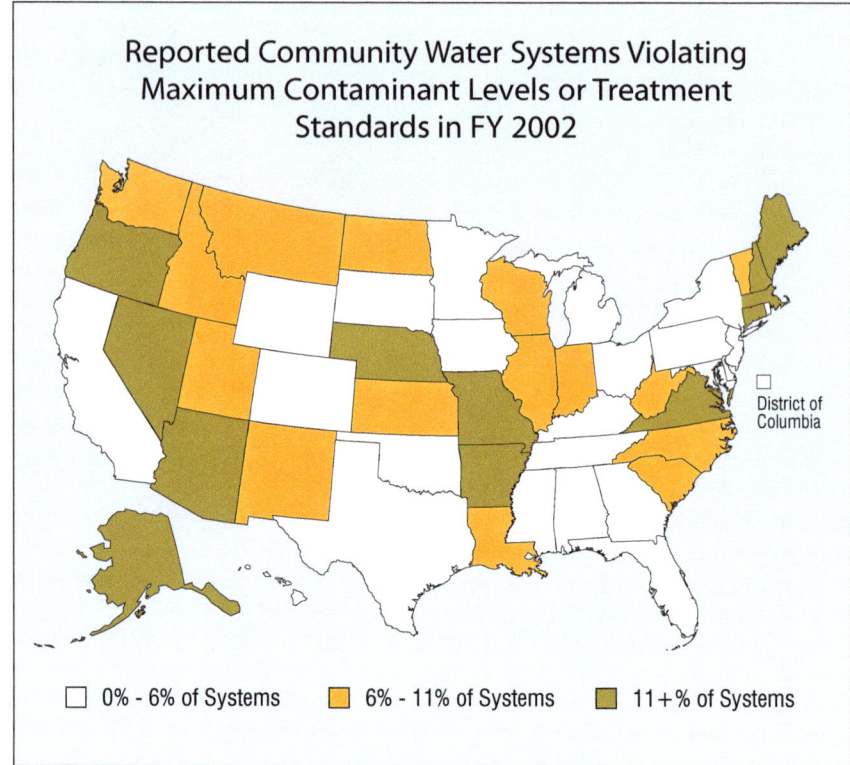

Reported Community Water Systems Violating Maximum Contaminant Levels or Treatment Standards in FY 2002

District of Columbia

☐ 0% - 6% of Systems ☐ 6% - 11% of Systems ☐ 11+% of Systems

Common Sources of Pollution

Naturally Occurring: microorganisms (wildlife and soils), radionuclides (underlying rock), nitrates and nitrites (nitrogen compounds in the soil), heavy metals (underground rocks containing arsenic, cadmium, chromium, lead, and selenium), fluoride.

Human Activities: bacteria and nitrates (human and animal wastes—septic tanks and large farms), heavy metals (mining construction, older fruit orchards), fertilizers and pesticides (used by you and others (anywhere crops or lawns are maintained)), industrial products and wastes (local factories, industrial plants, gas stations, dry cleaners, leaking underground storage tanks, landfills, and waste dumps), household wastes (cleaning solvents, used motor oil, paint, paint thinner), lead and copper (household plumbing materials), water treatment chemicals (wastewater treatment plants).

Nevertheless, problems with local drinking water can, and do, occur.

What Problems Can Occur?

Actual events of drinking water contamination are rare, and typically do not occur at levels likely to pose health concerns. However, as development in our modern society increases, there are growing numbers of activities that can contaminate our drinking water. Improperly disposed-of chemicals, animal and human wastes, wastes injected underground, and naturally occurring substances have the potential to contaminate drinking water. Likewise, drinking water that is not properly treated or disinfected, or that travels through an improperly maintained distribution system, may also pose a health risk. Greater vigilance by you, your water supplier, and your government can help prevent such events in your water supply.

Contaminants can enter water supplies either as a result of human and animal activities, or because they occur naturally in the environment. Threats to your drinking water may exist in your neighborhood, or may occur many miles away. For more information on drinking water threats, see *www.epa.gov/safewater/*

publicoutreach/landscapeposter.html. Some typical examples are microbial contamination, chemical contamination from fertilizers, and lead contamination.

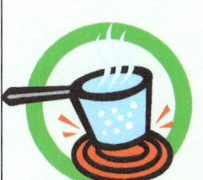

Boil Water Notices for Microbial Contaminants

When microorganisms such as those that indicate fecal contamination are found in drinking water, water suppliers are required to issue "Boil Water Notices." Boiling water for one minute kills the microorganisms that cause disease. Therefore, these notices serve as a precaution to the public. www.epa.gov/safewater/faq/emerg.html

Microbial Contamination:

The potential for health problems from microbial-contaminated drinking water is demonstrated by localized outbreaks of waterborne disease. Many of these outbreaks have been linked to contamination by bacteria or viruses, probably from human or animal wastes. For example, in 1999 and 2000, there were 39 reported disease outbreaks associated with drinking water, some of which were linked to public drinking water supplies.[5]

Certain **pathogens** (disease-causing **microorganisms**), such as *Cryptosporidium*, may occasionally pass through water filtration and disinfection processes in numbers high enough to cause health problems, particularly in vulnerable members of the population. *Cryptosporidium* causes the gastrointestinal disease, cryptosporidiosis, and can cause serious, sometimes fatal, symptoms, especially among sensitive members of the population. (See box on Sensitive Subpopulations on page 1.) A serious outbreak of cryptosporidiosis occurred in 1993 in Milwaukee, Wisconsin, causing more than 400,000 persons to be infected with the disease, and resulting in at least 50 deaths. This was the largest recorded outbreak of waterborne disease in United States history.[6]

Excessive levels of nitrates can cause "blue baby syndrome," which can be fatal without immediate medical attention.

Chemical Contamination From Fertilizers:

Nitrate, a chemical most commonly used as a fertilizer, poses an immediate threat to infants when it is found in drinking water at levels above the national standard. Nitrates are converted to nitrites in the intestines. Once absorbed into the bloodstream, nitrites prevent hemoglobin from transporting oxygen. (Older children have an enzyme that restores hemoglobin.) Excessive levels can cause "blue baby syndrome," which can be fatal without immediate medical attention. Infants most at risk for blue baby syndrome are those who are already sick, and while they are sick, consume food that is high in nitrates or drink water or formula mixed with water that is high in nitrates. Avoid using water with high nitrate levels for drinking. This is especially important for infants and young children, nursing mothers, pregnant women and certain elderly people.

Nitrates: Do NOT Boil

Do NOT boil water to attempt to reduce nitrates. Boiling water contaminated with nitrates increases its concentration and potential risk. If you are concerned about nitrates, talk to your health care provider about alternatives to boiling water for baby formula.

Lead Contamination:

Lead, a metal found in natural deposits, is commonly used in household plumbing materials and water service lines. The greatest exposure to lead is swallowing lead paint chips or breathing in lead dust. But lead in drinking water can also cause a variety of adverse health effects. In babies and children, exposure to lead in drinking water above the **action level** of lead (0.015 milligram per liter) can result in delays in physical and mental development, along with slight deficits in attention span and learning abilities. Adults who drink this water over many years could develop kidney problems or high blood pressure. Lead is rarely found in source water, but enters tap water through corrosion of plumbing materials. Very old and poorly maintained homes may be more likely to have lead pipes, joints, and solder. However, new homes are also at risk: pipes legally considered to be "lead-free" may contain up to eight percent lead. These pipes can leach significant amounts of lead in the water for the first several months after their installation. For more information on lead contamination, see *www.epa.gov/safewater/contaminants/dw_contamfs/lead.html.*

Lead: Do NOT Boil

Do NOT boil water to attempt to reduce lead. Boiling water increases lead concentration. Always use water from the cold tap for preparing baby formula, cooking, and drinking. Flush pipes first by running the water before using it. Allow the water to run until it's cold. If you have high lead levels in your tap water, talk to your health care provider about alternatives to using boiled water in baby formula.

For more information on drinking water contaminants that are regulated by EPA, see Appendix A, or visit *www.epa.gov/safewater/mcl.html.*

Where Can I Find More Information About My Drinking Water?

Drinking water varies from place to place, depending on the water's source and the treatment it receives. If your drinking water comes from a community water system, the system will deliver to its customers annual drinking water quality reports (or Consumer Confidence Reports). These reports will tell consumers what contaminants have been detected in their drinking water, how these detection levels compare to drinking water standards, and where their water comes from. The reports must be provided annually before July 1, and, in most cases, are mailed directly to customers' homes. Contact your water supplier to get a copy of your report, or see if your report is posted online at *www.epa.gov/safewater/dwinfo.htm.* Your state's department of health or environment can also be a valuable source of information. For help in locating these agencies, call the Safe Drinking Water Hotline. Further resources can be found in Appendix C. Information on testing household wells is on page 19.

---

[1] *Factoids: Drinking Water & Ground Water Statistics for 2002, 2003.*

[2] *Community Water Systems Survey 2000, Volume I, 2001.*

[3] *The Clean Water and Drinking Water Infrastructure Gap Analysis,* EPA 816-R-02-020.

[4] *Factoids: Drinking Water and Ground Water Statistics for 2001,* EPA 816-K-02-004.

[5] *Morbidity and Mortality Weekly Report: Surveillance for Waterborne Disease Outbreaks, United States 1999-2000, 2002.*

[6] *25 Years of the Safe Drinking Water Act, 1999.*

3. Where Does My Drinking Water Come From And How Is It Treated?

Your drinking water comes from **surface water** or **ground water**. The water that systems pump and treat from sources open to the atmosphere, such as rivers, lakes, and reservoirs is known as surface water. Water pumped from wells drilled into underground **aquifers**, geologic formations containing water, is called ground water. The quantity of water produced by a well depends on the nature of the rock, sand, or soil in the aquifer from which the water is drawn. Drinking water wells may be shallow (50 feet or less) or deep (more than 1,000 feet). More water systems have ground water than surface water as a source (approx. 147,000 v. 14,500), but more people drink from a surface water system (195 million v. 101,400). Large-scale water supply systems tend to rely on surface water resources, while smaller water systems tend to use ground water. Your water utility or public works department can tell you the source of your public water supply.

How Does Water Get To My Faucet?

An underground network of pipes typically delivers drinking water to the homes and businesses served by the water system. Small systems serving just a handful of households may be relatively simple, while large metropolitan systems can be extremely complex—sometimes consisting of thousands of miles of pipes serving millions of people. Drinking water must meet required health standards when it leaves the treatment plant. After treated water leaves the plant, it is monitored within the distribution system to identify and remedy any problems such as water main breaks, pressure variations, or growth of microorganisms.

How Is My Water Treated To Make It Safe?

Water utilities treat nearly 34 billion gallons of water every day.[1] The amount and type of treatment applied varies with the source and quality of the water. Generally, surface water systems require more treatment than ground water systems because they are directly exposed to the atmosphere and runoff from rain and melting snow.

Water suppliers use a variety of treatment processes to remove contaminants from drinking water. These individual processes can be arranged in a "treatment train" (a series of processes applied in a sequence). The most commonly used processes include coagulation (flocculation and sedimentation), filtration, and disinfection. Some water systems also use ion exchange and adsorption. Water utilities select the treatment combination most appropriate to treat the contaminants found in the **source water** of that particular system.

Coagulation (Flocculation & Sedimentation):

Flocculation: This step removes dirt and other particles suspended in the water. Alum and iron salts or synthetic organic polymers are added to the water to form tiny sticky particles called "floc," which attract the dirt particles.

> All sources of drinking water contain some naturally occurring contaminants. At low levels, these contaminants generally are not harmful in our drinking water. Removing all contaminants would be extremely expensive, and in most cases, would not provide increased protection of public health. A few naturally occurring minerals may actually improve the taste of drinking water and may even have nutritional value at low levels.

Sedimentation: The flocculated particles then settle naturally out of the water.

Filtration:

Many water treatment facilities use filtration to remove all particles from the water. Those particles include clays and silts, natural organic matter, precipitates from other treatment processes in the facility, iron and manganese, and microorganisms. Filtration clarifies the water and enhances the effectiveness of disinfection.

Water Treatment Plant

Follow a drop of water from the source through the treatment process. Water may be treated differently in different communities depending on the quality of the water which enters the plant. Groundwater is located underground and typically requires less treatment than water from lakes, rivers, and streams.

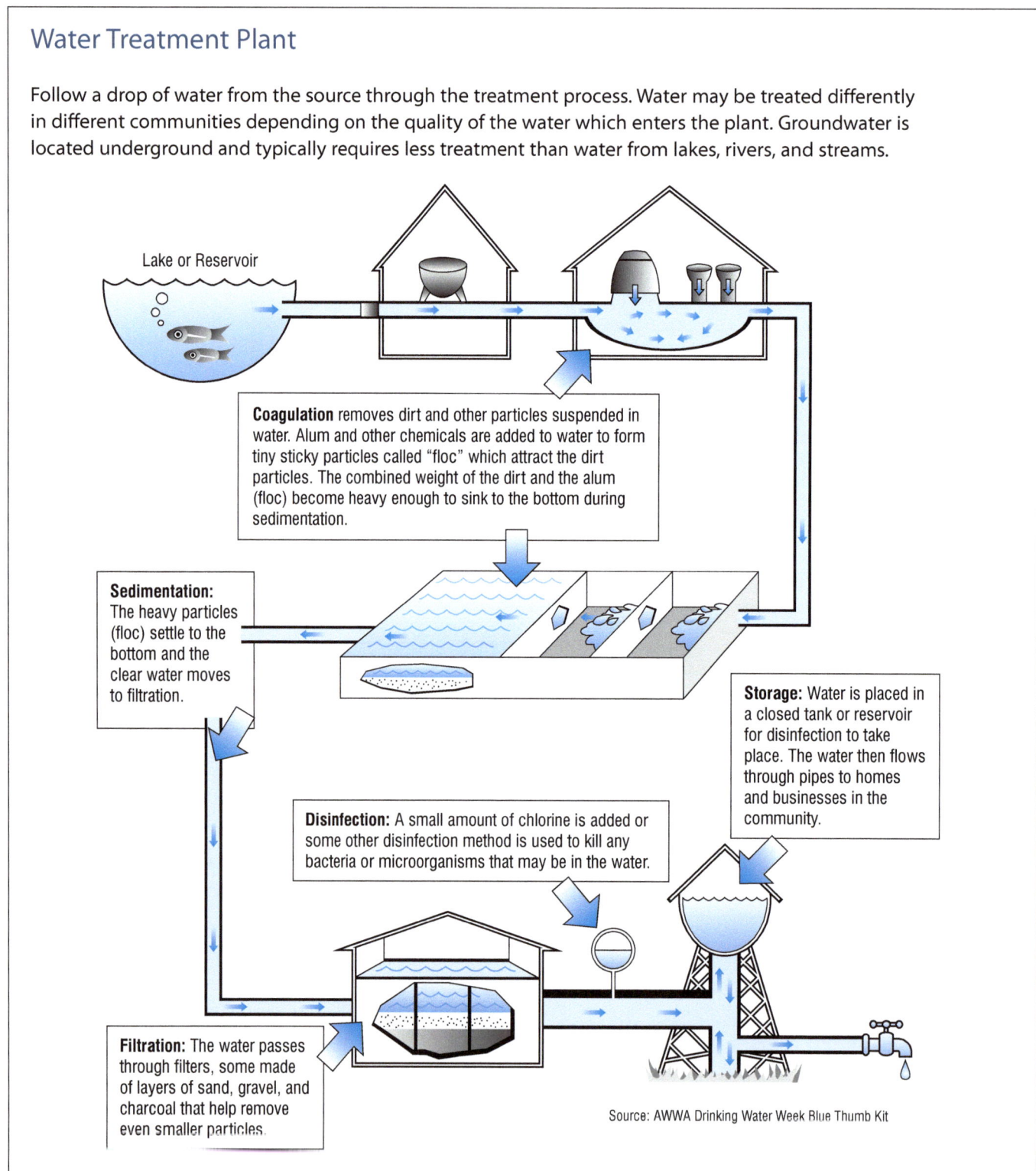

Lake or Reservoir

Coagulation removes dirt and other particles suspended in water. Alum and other chemicals are added to water to form tiny sticky particles called "floc" which attract the dirt particles. The combined weight of the dirt and the alum (floc) become heavy enough to sink to the bottom during sedimentation.

Sedimentation: The heavy particles (floc) settle to the bottom and the clear water moves to filtration.

Storage: Water is placed in a closed tank or reservoir for disinfection to take place. The water then flows through pipes to homes and businesses in the community.

Disinfection: A small amount of chlorine is added or some other disinfection method is used to kill any bacteria or microorganisms that may be in the water.

Filtration: The water passes through filters, some made of layers of sand, gravel, and charcoal that help remove even smaller particles.

Source: AWWA Drinking Water Week Blue Thumb Kit

Disinfection:

Disinfection of drinking water is considered to be one of the major public health advances of the 20th century. Water is often disinfected before it enters the distribution system to ensure that dangerous microbial contaminants are killed. Chlorine, chlorinates, or chlorine dioxides are most often used because they are very effective **disinfectants**, and residual concentrations can be maintained in the water system.

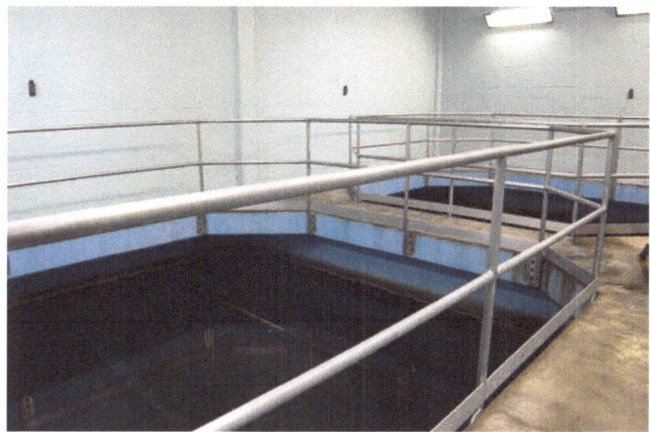

Water System Filtration Tank

Why Is My Water Bill Rising?

The cost of drinking water is rising as suppliers meet the needs of aging infrastructure, comply with public health standards, and expand service areas. In most cases, these increasing costs have caused water suppliers to raise their rates. However, despite rate increases, water is generally still a bargain compared to other utilities, such as electricity and phone service. In fact, in the United States, combined water and sewer bills average only about 0.5 percent of household income.[2]

---

[1] *Protect Your Drinking Water,* 2002.

[2] *Congressional Budget Office Study: Future Investment in Drinking Water & Wastewater Infrastructure, 2002.*

Disinfection Byproducts

Disinfection of drinking water is one of the major public health advances of the 20th century. However, sometimes the disinfectants themselves can react with naturally occurring materials in the water to form unintended byproducts, which may pose health risks. EPA recognizes the importance of removing microbial contaminants while simultaneously protecting the public from disinfection byproducts, and has developed regulations to limit the presence of these byproducts. For more information, see www.epa.gov/safewater/mdbp.html.

9

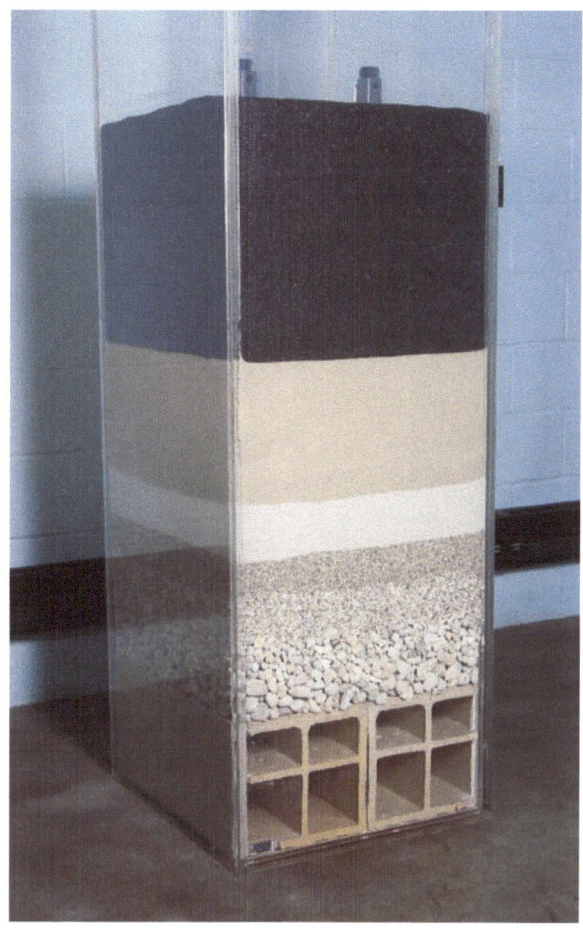

Water passes through charcoal, sand, and gravel layers in a water system's filtration tank.

4. How Do We Use Drinking Water In Our Homes?

We take our water supplies for granted, yet they are limited. Only one percent of all the world's water can be used for drinking. Nearly 97 percent of the world's water is salty or otherwise undrinkable, and the other two percent is locked away in ice caps and glaciers. There is no "new" water: whether our source water is a stream, river, lake, spring, or well, we are using the same water the dinosaurs used millions of years ago.

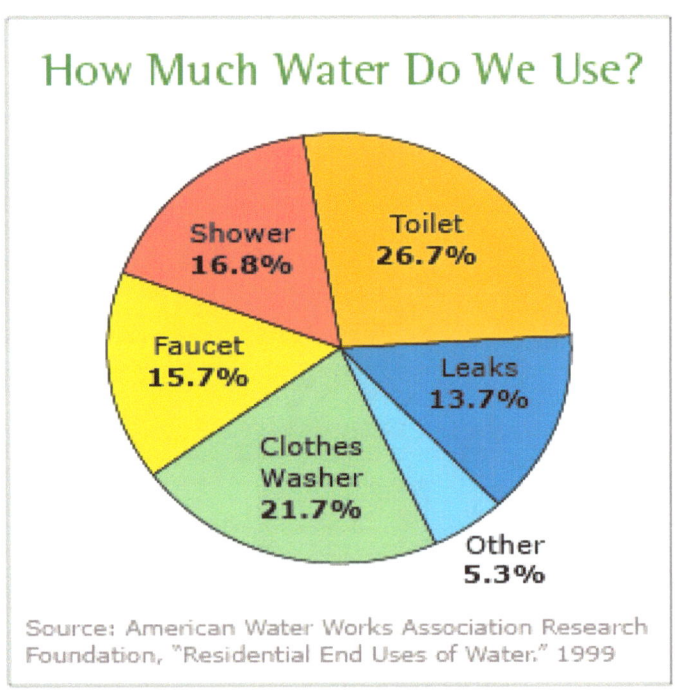

Source: American Water Works Association Research Foundation, "Residential End Uses of Water." 1999

The average American uses about 90 gallons of water each day in the home, and each American household uses approximately 107,000 gallons of water each year.[1] For the most part, we use water treated to meet drinking water standards to flush toilets, water lawns, and wash dishes, clothes, and cars. In fact, 50-70 percent of home water is used for watering lawns and gardens.[2] Nearly 14 percent of the water a typical homeowner pays for is never even used—it leaks down the drain.[3]

How Much Water Do Homes In The U.S. Use Compared To Other Countries?

Americans use much more water each day than individuals in both developed and undeveloped countries: For example, the average European uses 53 gallons; the average Sub-Saharan citizen, 3-5 gallons.[4]

Water efficiency plays an important role in protecting water sources and improving water quality. By using water wisely, we can save money and help the environment. Water efficiency means using less water to provide the same benefit. Using water-saving techniques could save you hundreds of dollars each year, while also reducing the amount of pollutants entering our waterways.

How Do Drinking Water Utilities Conserve Water?

Water utilities forecast water source availability, growth in population, and water demand to ensure adequate future water supplies during normal conditions, as well as periods of drought. When water shortages are predicted or experienced, water utilities have many options for conserving water. Temporary cutbacks or permanent operating adjustments can help conserve water.

Temporary cutbacks may include:

* Reduction of system-wide operating pressure, and

* Water use bans, restrictions, and rationing.

Permanent conservation measures may include:

- Subsidizing use of water-efficient faucets, toilets, and showerheads,
- Public education and voluntary use reduction,
- Billing practices that impose higher rates for higher amounts of water use,
- Building codes that require water-efficient fixtures and appliances,
- Leak detection surveys and meter testing, repair, and replacement, and
- Reduction in use and increase in recycling of industrial water.

How Can Businesses Conserve Water?

The industrial and commercial sectors can conserve water through recycling and waste reduction. Industry has implemented conservation measures to comply with state and federal water pollution controls. Evaluation of industrial plant data may show that a particular process or manufacturing step uses the most water or causes the greatest contamination. Such areas can be targeted for water conservation. Also, water that is contaminated by one process may be usable in other plant processes that do not require high-quality water.

How Can I Conserve Water?

The national average cost of water is $2.00 per 1,000 gallons. The average American family spends about $474 each year on water and sewage charges.[5] American households spend an additional $230 per year on water heating costs.[6] By replacing appliances such as the dishwasher and inefficient fixtures such as toilets and showerheads, you can save a substantial amount each year in water, sewage, and energy costs.

There are many ways to save water in and around your home. Here are the five that might get the best results:

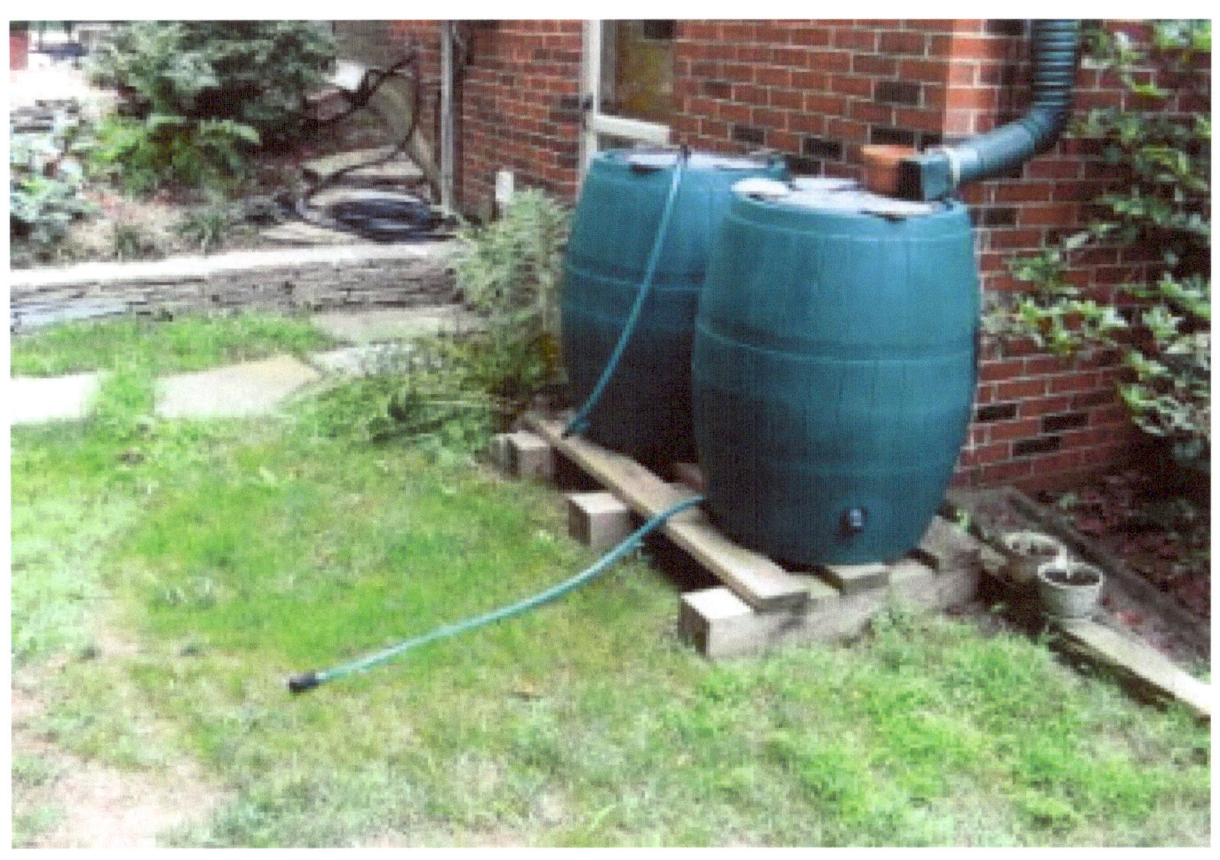

- *Stop Leaks.*
- *Replace Old Toilets* with models that use 1.6 gallons or less per flush.
- *Replace Old Clothes Washers* with EPA Energy Star certified models.
- *Plant the Right Kind of Garden* that requires less water.
- *Provide Only the Water Plants Need.*

For more information on ways to conserve water in the home, see *www.epa.gov/water/waterefficiency.html* or *www.h2ouse.org.*

[1] *Water Trivia Facts,* EPA 80-F-95-001.
[2] AWWA *Stats on Tap.*
[3] *Using Water Wisely in the Home,* 2002.
[4] *The Use of Water Today,* World Water Council.
[5] *Investing in America's Water Infrastructure,* 2002.
[6] *Using Water Wisely in the Home,* 2002.

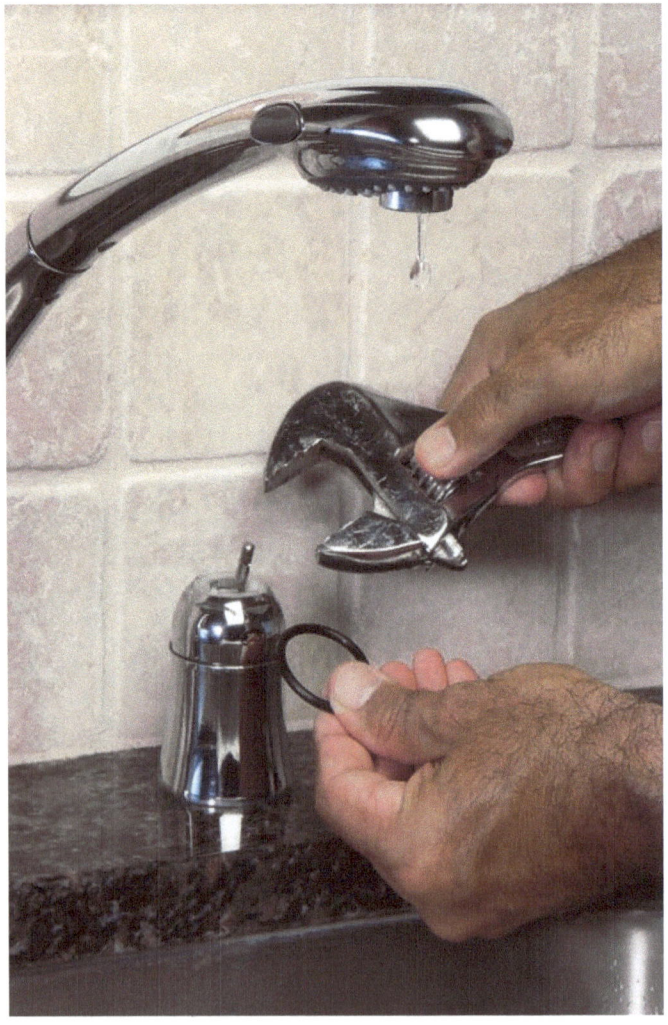

Nearly 14 percent of the water a typical homeowner pays for is never even used— it leaks down the drain.

Using Water Wisely in the Home, 2002

5. What's Being Done To Improve Water Security?

What Security Measures Are In Place To Protect Water Systems?

Drinking water utilities today find themselves facing new responsibilities due to concerns over water system security and counter-terrorism. EPA is committed to the safety of public drinking water supplies and has taken numerous steps to work with utilities, other government agencies, and law enforcement to minimize threats.

The Public Health Security and Bioterrorism Preparedness and Response Act of 2002 requires that all community water systems serving more than 3,300 people evaluate their susceptibility to potential threats and identify corrective actions. EPA has provided assistance to help utilities with these **Vulnerability Assessments** by giving direct grants to large systems, supporting self-assessment tools, and providing technical help and training to small and medium utilities. For more information on water system security, see *www.epa.gov/safewater/security.*

How Can I Help Protect My Drinking Water?

Local drinking water and wastewater systems may be targets for terrorists and other would-be criminals

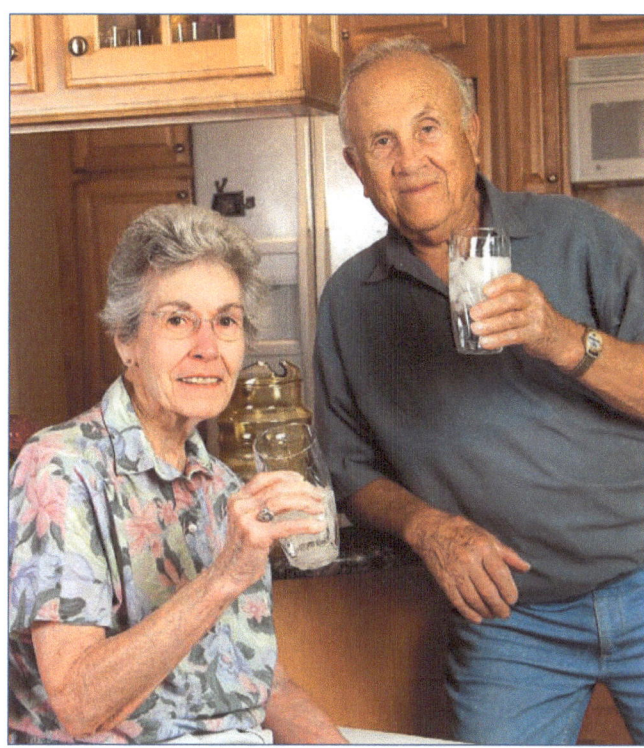

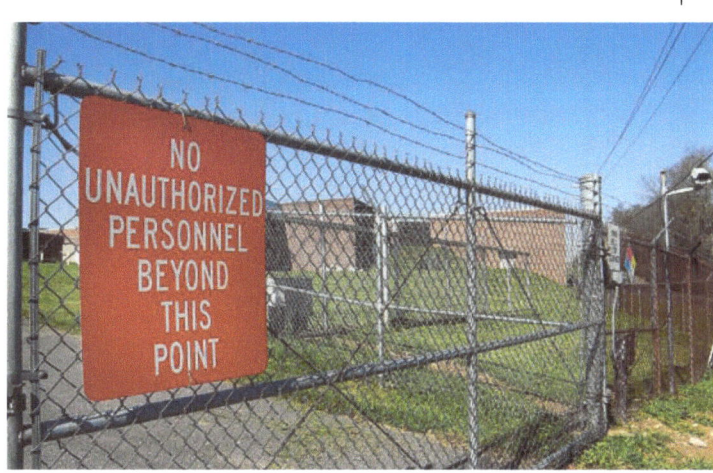

wishing to disrupt and cause harm to your community water supplies or wastewater facilities.

Because utilities are often located in isolated areas, drinking water sources and wastewater collection systems may cover large areas that are difficult to secure and patrol. Residents can be educated to notice and report any suspicious activity in and around local water utilities. Any residents interested in protecting their water resources and community as a whole can join together with law enforcement, neighborhood watch groups, water suppliers, wastewater operators, and other local public health officials. If you witness suspicious activities, report them to your local law enforcement authorities.

Examples of suspicious activity might include:

- People climbing or cutting a utility fence

- People dumping or discharging material to a water reservoir

- Unidentified truck or car parked or loitering near waterway or facilities for no apparent reason

- Suspicious opening or tampering with manhole covers, fire hydrants, buildings, or equipment

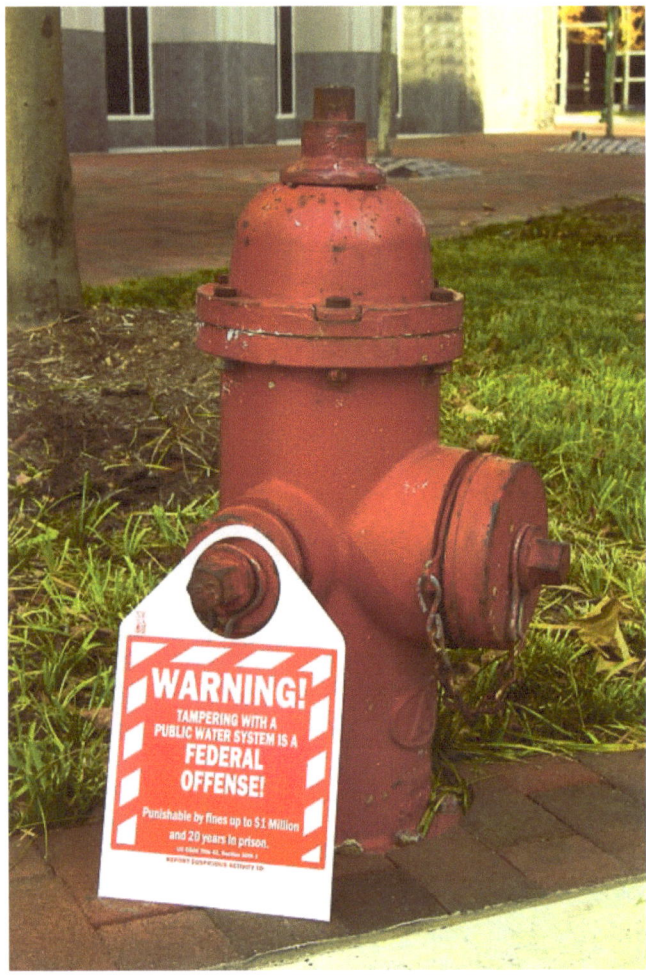

- People climbing or on top of water tanks

- People photographing or videotaping utility facilities, structures or equipment

- Strangers hanging around locks or gates

Report suspicious activity to local authorities

Do not confront strangers. Instead report suspicious activities to local authorities.

When reporting an incident:

- State the nature of the incident

- Identify yourself and your location

- Identify location of activity

- Describe any vehicle involved (color, make, model, plate number)

- Describe the participants (how many, sex, race, color of hair, height, weight, clothing)

For emergencies, dial 9-1-1 or other local emergency response numbers.

For more information on water security, visit: *www.epa.gov/safewater/security*

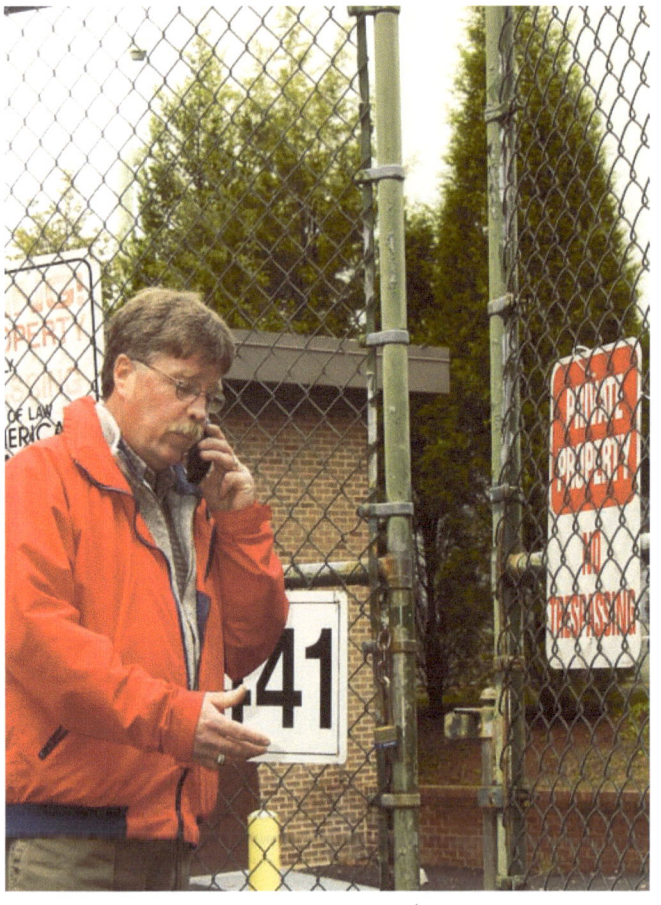

Safe Drinking Water Hotline: 800-426-4791

6. What Can I Do If There Is A Problem With My Drinking Water?

Local incidents, such as spills and treatment problems, can lead to short-term needs for alternative water supplies or in-home water treatment. In isolated cases, individuals may need to rely on alternative sources for the long term, due to their individual health needs or problems with obtaining new drinking water supplies.

What Alternative Sources Of Water Are Available?

Bottled water is sold in supermarkets and convenience stores. Some companies lease or sell water dispensers or bubblers and regularly deliver large bottles of water to homes and businesses. It is expensive compared to water from a public water system. The bottled water quality varies among brands, because of the variations in the source water used, costs, and company practices.

The U.S. Food and Drug Administration (FDA) regulates bottled water used for drinking. While most consumers assume that bottled water is at least as safe as tap water, there are still potential risks. Although required to meet the same safety standards as public water supplies, bottled water does not undergo the same testing and reporting as water from a treatment facility. Water that is bottled and sold in the same state may not be subject to any federal standards at all. Those with compromised immune systems may want to read bottled water labels to make sure more stringent treatments have been used, such as reverse osmosis, distillation, UV radiation, or filtration by an absolute 1 micron filter.

Check with NSF International to see if your bottled water adheres to FDA and international drinking water standards. The International Bottled Water Association can also provide information on which brands adhere to even more stringent requirements. Contact information is listed in Appendix C.

Can I Do Anything In My House To Improve The Safety Of My Drinking Water?

Most people do not need to treat drinking water in their home to make it safe. However, a home water treatment unit can improve water's taste, or provide a factor of safety for those people more vulnerable to waterborne disease. There are different options for home treatment systems. Point-of-use (POU) systems treat water at a single tap. Point-of-entry (POE) systems treat water used throughout the house. POU systems can be installed in various places in the home, including the counter top, the faucet itself, or under the sink. POE systems are installed where the water line enters the house.

POU and POE devices are based on various contaminant removal technologies. Filtration, ion exchange, reverse osmosis, and distillation are some of the treatment methods used. All types of units are generally available from retailers, or by mail order. Prices can reach well into the hundreds and sometimes thousands of dollars, and depending on the method and location of installation, plumbing can also add to the cost.

TREATMENT DEVICE	WHAT IT DOES TO WATER	TREATMENT LIMITATIONS
Activated Carbon Filter (includes mixed media that remove heavy metals)	√ Adsorbs organic contaminants that cause taste and odor problems. √ Somedesigns remove chlorination byproducts; √ Some types remove cleaning solvents and pesticides	Is efficient in removing metals such as lead and copper Does not remove nitrate, bacteria or dissolved minerals
Ion Exchange Unit (with activated alumina)	√ Removes minerals, particularly calcium and magnesium that make water "hard" √ Some designs remove radium and barium √ Removes fluoride	If water has oxidized iron or iron bacteria, the ion-exchange resin will become coated or clogged and lose its softening ability
Reverse Osmosis Unit (with carbon)	√ Removes nitrates, sodium, other dissolved inorganics and organic compounds √ Removes foul tastes, smells or colors √ May also reduce the level of some pesticides, dioxins and chloroform and petrochemicals	Does not remove all inorganic and organic contaminants
Distillation Unit	√ Removes nitrates, bacteria, sodium, hardness, dissolved solids, most organic compounds, heavy metals, and radionucleides √ Kills bacteria	Does not remove some volatile organic contaminants, certain pesticides and volatile solvents Bacteria may recolonize on the cooling coils during inactive periods

Activated carbon filters adsorb **organic contaminants** that cause taste and odor problems. Depending on their design, some units can remove chlorination byproducts, some cleaning solvents, and pesticides. To maintain the effectiveness of these units, the carbon canisters must be replaced periodically. Activated carbon filters are efficient in removing metals such as lead and copper if they are designed to absorb or remove lead.

Because ion exchange units can be used to remove minerals from your water, particularly calcium and magnesium, they are sold for water softening. Some ion exchange softening units remove radium and barium from water. Ion exchange systems that employ activated alumina are used to remove fluoride and arsenate from water. These units must be regenerated periodically with salt.

Reverse osmosis treatment units generally remove a more diverse list of contaminants than other systems. They can remove nitrates, sodium, other dissolved inorganics, and organic compounds.

Distillation units boil water and condense the resulting steam to create distilled water. Depending on their design, some of these units may allow vaporized organic contaminants to condense back into the product water, thus minimizing the removal of organics.

You may choose to boil your water to remove microbial contaminants. Keep in mind that boiling reduces the volume of water by about 20 percent, thus concentrating those contaminants not affected by the temperature of boiling water, such as nitrates and

pesticides. For more information on boiling water, see page 5 of this booklet.

No one unit can remove everything. Have your water tested by a certified laboratory prior to purchasing any device. Do not rely on the tests conducted by salespeople that want to sell you their product.

Where Can I Learn More About Home Treatment Systems?

Your local library has articles, such as those found in consumer magazines, on the effectiveness of these devices.

The U.S. General Accounting Office published a booklet called *Drinking Water: Inadequate Regulation of Home Treatment Units Leaves Consumers At Risk* (December 1991). To read this booklet, visit *www.gao.gov* and search for **document number RCED-92-34**, or call (202) 512-6000.

Maintaining Treatment Devices

All POU and POE treatment units need maintenance to operate effectively. If they are not maintained properly, contaminants may accumulate in the units and actually make your water worse. In addition, some vendors may make claims about their effectiveness that have no merit. Units are tested for their safety and effectiveness by two organizations, NSF International and Underwriters Laboratory. In addition, the Water Quality Association represents the household, commercial, industrial and small community treatment industry and can help you locate a professional that meets their code of ethics. EPA does not test or certify these treatment units.

This treatment device is for point of use (POU). For more information on different types of devices contact NSF International, Underwriters Laboratory, or the Water Quality Association See Appendix C for contact information.

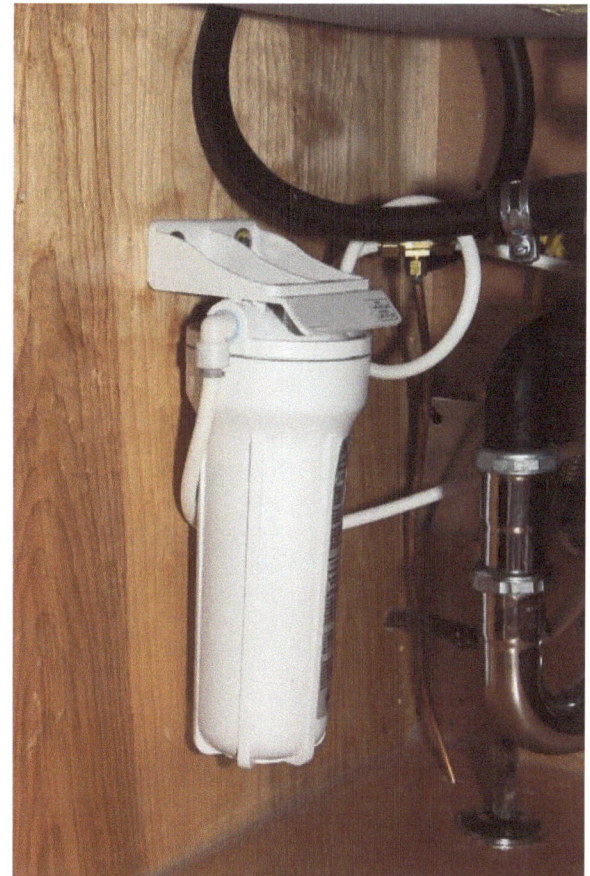

7. How Safe Is The Drinking Water In My Household Well?

EPA regulates public water systems; it does not have the authority to regulate private wells. Approximately 15 percent of Americans rely on their own private drinking water supplies (*Drinking Water from Household Wells*, 2002), and these supplies are not subject to EPA standards. Unlike public drinking water systems serving many people, they do not have experts regularly checking the water's source and its quality before it is sent to the tap. These households must take special precautions to ensure the protection and maintenance of their drinking water supplies.

Drinking Water from Household Wells is an EPA publication available to specifically address special concerns of a private drinking water supply. To learn more, or to obtain a copy, visit *www.epa.gov/safewater/ privatewells,* or call the Safe Drinking Water Hotline.

How Much Risk Can I Expect?

The risk of having problems depends on how good your well is—how well it was built and located, and how well you maintain it. It also depends on your local environment. That includes the quality of the aquifer from which your water is drawn and the human activities going on in your area that can affect your well.

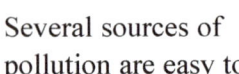

Several sources of pollution are easy to spot by sight, taste, or smell. However, many serious problems can be found only by testing your water. Knowing the possible threats in your area will help you decide the kind of tests you may need.

What Should I Do?

There are six basic steps you can take to help protect your private drinking water supply:

1. Identify potential problem sources.

2. Talk with local experts.

3. Have your water tested periodically.

4. Have the test results interpreted and explained clearly.

5. Set and follow a regular maintenance schedule for your well, and keep up-to-date records.

6. Immediately remedy any problems.

Identify Potential Problem Sources

Understanding and spotting possible pollution sources is the first step to safeguarding your drinking water. If your drinking water comes from a well, you may also have a **septic system**. Septic systems and other on-site wastewater disposal systems are major potential sources of contamination of private water supplies if they are poorly maintained or located improperly, or if they are used for disposal of toxic chemicals. Information on septic systems is available from local health departments, state agencies, and the National Small Flows Clearinghouse *(www.epa.gov/owm/ mab/smcomm/nsfc.htm)* at (800) 624-8301. A septic system design manual and guidance on system maintenance are available from EPA (*www.epa.gov/ OW-OWM.html/mtb/decent/homeowner.htm*).

Talk With Local Experts

Ground water conditions vary greatly from place to place, and local experts can give you the best information about your drinking water supply. Some examples are your health department's "sanitarian," local water-well contractors, public water system officials, county extension agents of the Natural Resources Conservation Service (NRCS), local or county planning commissions, and your local library.

Have Your Water Tested Periodically

Test your water every year for total **coliform** bacteria, nitrates, total dissolved solids, and pH levels. If you suspect other contaminants, test for these as well. As the tests can be expensive, limit them to possible problems specific to your situation. Local experts can help you identify these contaminants. You should also test your water after replacing or repairing any part of the system, or if you notice any change in your water's look, taste, or smell.

Often, county health departments perform tests for bacteria and nitrates. For other substances, health departments, environmental offices, or county governments should have a list of state-certified laboratories. Your State Laboratory Certification Officer can also provide you with this list. Call the Safe Drinking Water Hotline for the name and number of your state's certification officer. Any laboratory you use should be certified to do drinking water testing.

Have Your Test Results Interpreted And Explained Clearly

Compare your well's test results to federal and state drinking water standards (see Appendix A, or visit *www.epa.gov/safewater/mcl.html* or call the Safe Drinking Water Hotline). You may need to consult experts to aid you in understanding your results, such as the state agency that licenses water well contractors, your local health department, or your state's drinking water program.

Protecting Your Ground Water Supply

- Periodically inspect exposed parts of the well for problems such as:
  - Cracked, corroded, or damaged well casing
  - Broken or missing well cap
  - Settling and cracking of surface seals.
- Slope the area around the well to drain surface runoff away from the well.
- Install a well cap or sanitary seal to prevent unauthorized use of, or entry into, the well.
- Disinfect drinking water wells at least once per year with bleach or hypochlorite granules, according to the manufacturer's directions.
- Have the well tested once a year for coliform bacteria, nitrates, and other constituents of concern.
- Keep accurate records of any well maintenance, such as disinfection or sediment removal, that may require the use of chemicals in the well.
- Hire a certified well driller for any new well construction, modification, or abandonment and closure.
- Avoid mixing or using pesticides, fertilizers, herbicides, degreasers, fuels, and other pollutants near the well.
- Do not dispose of wastes in dry wells or in abandoned wells.
- Do not cut off the well casing below the land surface.
- Pump and inspect septic systems as often as recommended by your local health department.
- Never dispose of hazardous materials in a septic system.

19

Set A Regular Maintenance Schedule For Your Well And Your Septic System

Proper well and septic system construction and continued maintenance are keys to the safety of your water supply. Your state water well and septic system contractor licensing agency, local health department, or local public water system professional can provide information on well construction. Make certain your contractors are licensed by the state, if required, or certified by the National Ground Water Association.

Maintain your well, fixing problems before they reach crisis levels, and keep up-to-date records of well installation and repairs, as well as plumbing and water costs. Protect your own well area from contamination.

Immediately Remedy Any Problems

If you find that your well water is contaminated, fix the problem as soon as possible. Consider connecting into a nearby community water system, if one is available. You may want to install a water treatment device to remove impurities. Information on these devices is provided on page 16. If you connect to a public water system, remember to close your well properly.

After A Flood-Concerns And Advisories

- Stay away from well pump to avoid electric shock.

- Do not drink or wash from a flooded well.

- Pump the well until water runs clear.

- If water does not run clear, contact the county or state health department or extension service for advice.

Animal waste

can

contaminate

your

water supply

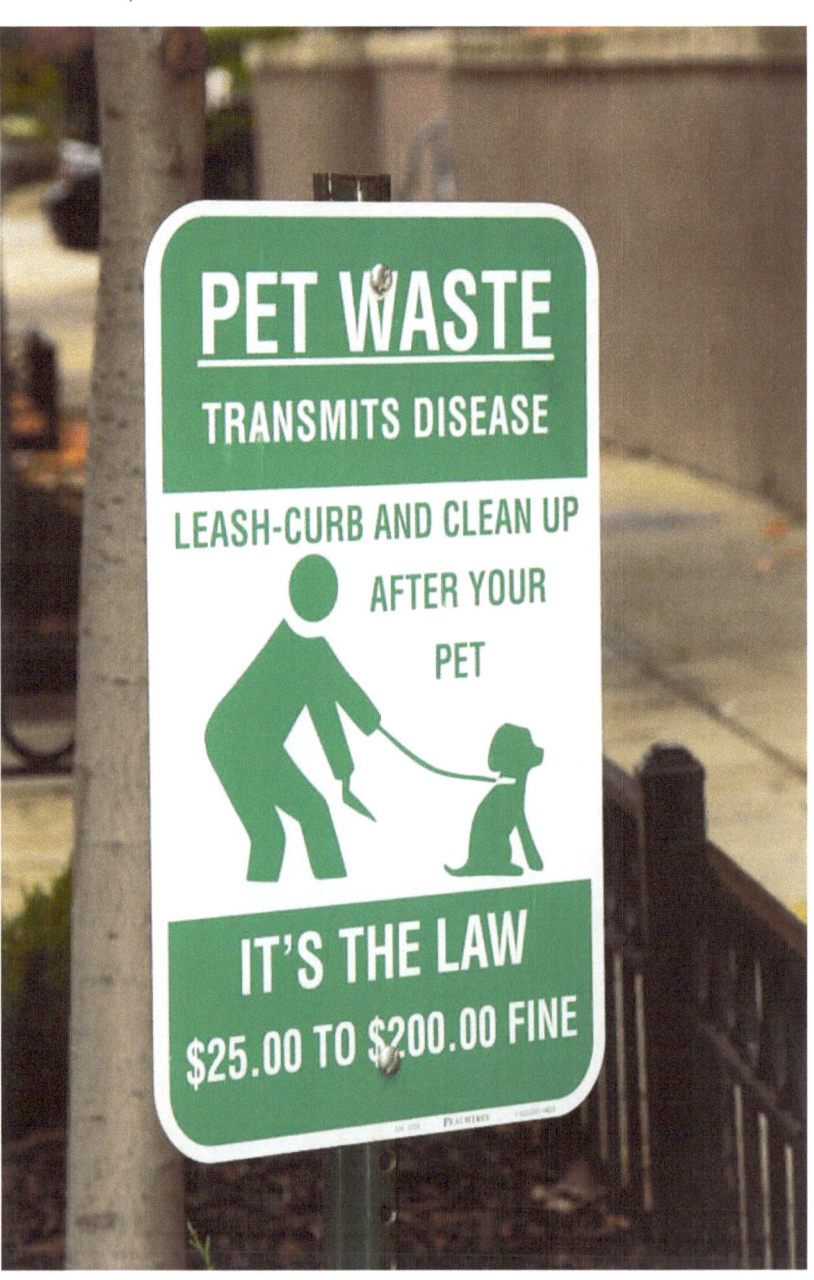

20

8. What You Can Do To Protect Your Drinking Water

Drinking water protection is a shared responsibility. Many actions are underway to protect our nation's drinking water, and there are many opportunities for citizens to become involved.

Be Involved!

EPA activities to protect drinking water include setting drinking water standards and overseeing the work of states that enforce federal standards—or stricter ones set by the individual state. EPA holds many public meetings on issues ranging from proposed drinking water standards to the development of databases. You can also comment on proposed drafts of other upcoming EPA documents. A list of public meetings and regulations open for comment can be found at *www.epa.gov/safewater/pubinput/html.*

Be Informed!

- Read the annual Consumer Confidence Report provided by your water supplier. Some Consumer Confidence Reports are available at *www.epa.gov/safewater/dwinfo.htm.*

- Use information from your state's Source Water Assessment to learn about potential threats to your water source.

- If you are one of the 15 percent of Americans who uses a private source of drinking water—such as a well, cistern, or spring—find out what activities are taking place in your **watershed** that may impact your drinking water; talk to local experts/ test your water periodically; and maintain your well properly.

- Find out if the Clean Water Act standards for your drinking water source are intended to protect water for drinking, in addition to fishing and swimming.

Be Observant!

- Look around your watershed and look for announcements in the local media about activities that may pollute your drinking water.

- **Form and operate** a citizens watch network within your community to communicate regularly with law enforcement, your public water supplier and wastewater operator. **Communication** is key to a safer community!

- **Be alert**. Get to know your water/wastewater utilities, their vehicles, routines and their personnel.

- **Become aware of your surroundings**. This will help you to recognize suspicious activity as opposed to normal daily activities.

Other Ways To Get Involved

- Attend public hearings on new construction, storm water permitting, and town planning.

- Keep your public officials accountable by asking to see their environmental impact statements.

- Ask questions about any issue that may affect your water source.

- Participate with your government and your water system as they make funding decisions.

- Volunteer or help recruit volunteers to participate in your community's contaminant monitoring activities.

- Help ensure that local utilities that protect your water have adequate resources to do their job.

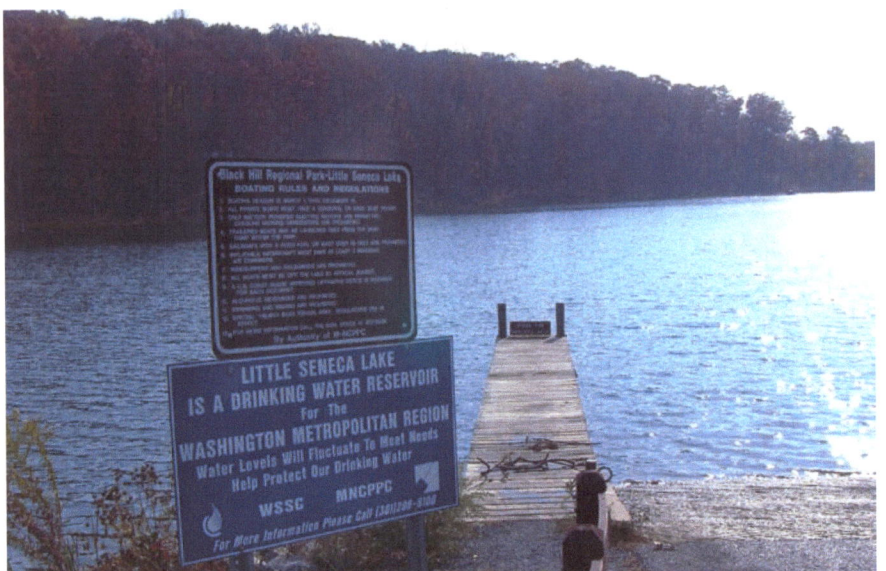

Don't Contaminate!

-     Reduce paved areas: use permeable surfaces that allow rain to soak through, not run off.

-     Reduce or eliminate pesticide application: test your soil before applying chemicals, and use plants that require little or no water, pesticides, or fertilizers.

-     Reduce the amount of trash you create: reuse and recycle.

-     Recycle used oil: 1 quart of oil can contaminate 2 million gallons of drinking water—take your used oil and antifreeze to a service station or recycling center.

- Take the bus instead of your car one day a week: you could prevent 33 pounds of carbon dioxide emissions each day.

- Keep pollutants away from boat marinas and waterways: keep boat motors well-tuned to prevent leaks, select nontoxic cleaning products and use a drop cloth, and clean and maintain boats away from the water.

For more information on how you can help protect your local drinking water source, call the Safe Drinking Water Hotline, or check *www.epa.gov/safewater/publicoutreach*. Additional resources are listed in Appendix C.

- If you see any suspicious activities in or around your water supply, please notify local authorities or call 9-1-1 immediately to report the incident.

Stormwater runoff threatens our sources of drinking water. As this water washes over roofs, pavement, farms and grassy areas, it picks up fertilizers, pesticides and litter, and deposits them in surface water and ground water. Here are some other threats to our drinking water:

Every year:

- We apply 67 million pounds of pesticides that contain toxic and harmful chemicals to our lawns.

- We produce more than 230 million tons of municipal solid water—approximately five pounds of trash or garbage per person per day—that contain bacteria, nitrates, viruses, synthetic detergents, and household chemicals.

- Our more than 12 million recreational and houseboats and 10,000 boat marinas release solvents, gasoline, detergents, and raw sewage directly into our rivers, lakes and streams.

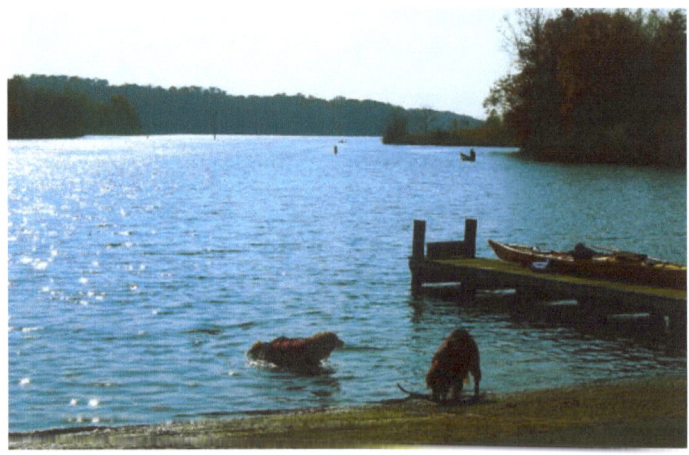

National Primary Drinking Water Regulations

	Contaminant	MCL or TT[1] (mg/L)[2]	Potential health effects from long-term[3] exposure above the MCL	Common sources of contaminant in drinking water	Public Health Goal (mg/L)[2]
OC	Acrylamide	TT[4]	Nervous system or blood problems; increased risk of cancer	Added to water during sewage/ wastewater treatment	zero
OC	Alachlor	0 002	Eye, liver, kidney or spleen problems; anemia; increased risk of cancer	Runoff from herbicide used on row crops	zero
R	Alpha/photon emitters	15 picocuries per Liter (pCi/L)	Increased risk of cancer	Erosion of natural deposits of certain minerals that are radioactive and may emit a form of radiation known as alpha radiation	zero
IOC	Antimony	0 006	Increase in blood cholesterol; decrease in blood sugar	Discharge from petroleum refineries; fir retardants; ceramics; electronics; solder	0 006
IOC	Arsenic	0 010	Skin damage or problems with circulatory systems, and may have increased risk of getting cancer	Erosion of natural deposits; runoff from orchards; runoff from glass & electronics production wastes	0
IOC	Asbestos (fiber >10 micrometers)	7 million fiber per Liter (MFL)	Increased risk of developing benign intestinal polyps	Decay of asbestos cement in water mains; erosion of natural deposits	7 MFL
OC	Atrazine	0 003	Cardiovascular system or reproductive problems	Runoff from herbicide used on row crops	0 003
IOC	Barium	2	Increase in blood pressure	Discharge of drilling wastes; discharge from metal refineries erosion of natural deposits	2
OC	Benzene	0 005	Anemia; decrease in blood platelets; increased risk of cancer	Discharge from factories; leaching from gas storage tanks and landfill	zero
OC	Benzo(a)pyrene (PAHs)	0 0002	Reproductive difficulties increased risk of cancer	Leaching from linings of water storage tanks and distribution lines	zero
IOC	Beryllium	0 004	Intestinal lesions	Discharge from metal refinerie and coal-burning factories; discharge from electrical, aerospace, and defense industries	0 004
R	Beta photon emitters	4 millirems per year	Increased risk of cancer	Decay of natural and man-made deposits of certain minerals that are radioactive and may emit forms of radiation known as photons and beta radiation	zero
DBP	Bromate	0 010	Increased risk of cancer	Byproduct of drinking water disinfection	zero
IOC	Cadmium	0 005	Kidney damage	Corrosion of galvanized pipes; erosion of natural deposits; discharge from metal refineries runoff from waste batteries and paints	0 005
OC	Carbofuran	0 04	Problems with blood, nervous system, or reproductive system	Leaching of soil fumigant used on rice and alfalfa	0 04
OC	Carbon tetrachloride	0 005	Liver problems; increased risk of cancer	Discharge from chemical plants and other industrial activities	zero
D	Chloramines (as Cl$_2$)	MRDL=4 0[1]	Eye/nose irritation; stomach discomfort; anemia	Water additive used to control microbes	MRDLG=4[1]
OC	Chlordane	0 002	Liver or nervous system problems; increased risk of cancer	Residue of banned termiticide	zero
D	Chlorine (as Cl$_2$)	MRDL=4 0[1]	Eye/nose irritation; stomach discomfort	Water additive used to control microbes	MRDLG=4[1]
D	Chlorine dioxide (as ClO$_2$)	MRDL=0 8[1]	Anemia; infants, young children, and fetuses of pregnant women: nervous system effects	Water additive used to control microbes	MRDLG=0 8[1]
DBP	Chlorite	1 0	Anemia; infants, young children, and fetuses of pregnant women: nervous system effects	Byproduct of drinking water disinfection	0 8
OC	Chlorobenzene	0 1	Liver or kidney problems	Discharge from chemical and agricultural chemical factories	0 1
IOC	Chromium (total)	0 1	Allergic dermatitis	Discharge from steel and pulp mills; erosion of natural deposits	0 1
IOC	Copper	TT[5]; Action Level = 1 3	Short-term exposure: Gastrointestinal distress Long-term exposure: Liver or kidney damage People with Wilson's Disease should consult their personal doctor if the amount of copper in their water exceeds the action level	Corrosion of household plumbing systems; erosion of natural deposits	1 3
M	*Cryptosporidium*	TT[7]	Short-term exposure: Gastrointestinal illness (e g , diarrhea, vomiting, cramps)	Human and animal fecal waste	zero

Safe Drinking Water Hotline: 800-426-4791

	Contaminant	MCL or TT[1] (mg/L)[2]	Potential health effects from long-term[3] exposure above the MCL	Common sources of contaminant in drinking water	Public Health Goal (mg/L)[2]
IOC	Cyanide (as free cyanide)	0 2	Nerve damage or thyroid problems	Discharge from steel/metal factories; discharge from plastic and fertilizer factories	0 2
OC	2,4-D	0 07	Kidney, liver, or adrenal gland problems	Runoff from herbicide used on row crops	0 07
OC	Dalapon	0 2	Minor kidney changes	Runoff from herbicide used on rights of way	0 2
OC	1,2-Dibromo-3-chloropropane (DBCP)	0 0002	Reproductive difficulties increased risk of cancer	Runoff/leaching from soil fumigant used on soybeans, cotton, pineapples, and orchards	zero
OC	o-Dichlorobenzene	0 6	Liver, kidney, or circulatory system problems	Discharge from industrial chemical factories	0 6
OC	p-Dichlorobenzene	0 075	Anemia; liver, kidney or spleen damage; changes in blood	Discharge from industrial chemical factories	0 075
OC	1,2-Dichloroethane	0 005	Increased risk of cancer	Discharge from industrial chemical factories	zero
OC	1,1-Dichloroethylene	0 007	Liver problems	Discharge from industrial chemical factories	0 007
OC	cis-1,2-Dichloroethylene	0 07	Liver problems	Discharge from industrial chemical factories	0 07
OC	trans-1,2-Dichloroethylene	0 1	Liver problems	Discharge from industrial chemical factories	0 1
OC	Dichloromethane	0 005	Liver problems; increased risk of cancer	Discharge from drug and chemical factories	zero
OC	1,2-Dichloropropane	0 005	Increased risk of cancer	Discharge from industrial chemical factories	zero
OC	Di(2-ethylhexyl) adipate	0 4	Weight loss, liver problems, or possible reproductive difficultie	Discharge from chemical factories	0 4
OC	Di(2-ethylhexyl) phthalate	0 006	Reproductive difficulties liver problems; increased risk of cancer	Discharge from rubber and chemical factories	zero
OC	Dinoseb	0 007	Reproductive difficulties	Runoff from herbicide used on soybeans and vegetables	0 007
OC	Dioxin (2,3,7,8-TCDD)	0 00000003	Reproductive difficulties increased risk of cancer	Emissions from waste incineration and other combustion; discharge from chemical factories	zero
OC	Diquat	0 02	Cataracts	Runoff from herbicide use	0 02
OC	Endothall	0 1	Stomach and intestinal problems	Runoff from herbicide use	0 1
OC	Endrin	0 002	Liver problems	Residue of banned insecticide	0 002
OC	Epichlorohydrin	TT[4]	Increased cancer risk; stomach problems	Discharge from industrial chemical factories; an impurity of some water treatment chemicals	zero
OC	Ethylbenzene	0 7	Liver or kidney problems	Discharge from petroleum refineries	0 7
OC	Ethylene dibromide	0 00005	Problems with liver, stomach, reproductive system, or kidneys; increased risk of cancer	Discharge from petroleum refineries	zero
M	Fecal coliform and *E. coli*	MCL[6]	Fecal coliforms and *E. coli* are bacteria whose presence indicates that the water may be contaminated with human or animal wastes Microbes in these wastes may cause short term effects, such as diarrhea, cramps, nausea, headaches, or other symptoms They may pose a special health risk for infants, young children, and people with severely compromised immune systems	Human and animal fecal waste	zero[6]
IOC	Fluoride	4 0	Bone disease (pain and tenderness of the bones); children may get mottled teeth	Water additive which promotes strong teeth; erosion of natural deposits; discharge from fertilizer and aluminum factories	4 0
M	*Giardia lamblia*	TT[7]	Short-term exposure: Gastrointestinal illness (e g , diarrhea, vomiting, cramps)	Human and animal fecal waste	zero
OC	Glyphosate	0 7	Kidney problems; reproductive difficultie	Runoff from herbicide use	0 7
DBP	Haloacetic acids (HAA5)	0 060	Increased risk of cancer	Byproduct of drinking water disinfection	n/a[9]
OC	Heptachlor	0 0004	Liver damage; increased risk of cancer	Residue of banned termiticide	zero
OC	Heptachlor epoxide	0 0002	Liver damage; increased risk of cancer	Breakdown of heptachlor	zero
M	Heterotrophic plate count (HPC)	TT[7]	HPC has no health effects; it is an analytic method used to measure the variety of bacteria that are common in water The lower the concentration of bacteria in drinking water, the better maintained the water system is	HPC measures a range of bacteria that are naturally present in the environment	n/a

LEGEND

D **Disinfectant**	IOC **Inorganic Chemical**	OC **Organic Chemical**
DBP **Disinfection Byproduct**	M **Microorganism**	R **Radionuclides**

Safe Drinking Water Hotline: 800-426-4791

Contaminant		MCL or TT[1] (mg/L)[2]	Potential health effects from long-term[3] exposure above the MCL	Common sources of contaminant in drinking water	Public Health Goal (mg/L)[2]
OC	Hexachlorobenzene	0 001	Liver or kidney problems; reproductive difficulties increased risk of cancer	Discharge from metal refinerie and agricultural chemical factories	zero
OC	Hexachlorocyclopentadiene	0 05	Kidney or stomach problems	Discharge from chemical factories	0 05
IOC	Lead	TT5; Action Level=0 015	Infants and children: Delays in physical or or mental development; children could show slight deficit in attention span and learning abilities; Adults: Kidney problems; high blood pressure	Corrosion of household plumbing systems; erosion of natural deposits	zero
M	*Legionella*	TT7	Legionnaire's Disease, a type of pneumonia	Found naturally in water; multiplies in heating systems	zero
OC	Lindane	0 0002	Liver or kidney problems	Runoff/leaching from insecticide used on cattle, lumber, gardens	0 0002
IOC	Mercury (inorganic)	0 002	Kidney damage	Erosion of natural deposits; discharge from refinerie and factories; runoff from landfill and croplands	0 002
OC	Methoxychlor	0 04	Reproductive difficulties	Runoff/leaching from insecticide used on fruits, vegetables, alfalfa, livestock	0 04
IOC	Nitrate (measured as Nitrogen)	10	Infants below the age of six months who drink water containing nitrate in excess of the MCL could become seriously ill and, if untreated, may die Symptoms include shortness of breath and blue-baby syndrome	Runoff from fertilizer use; leaching from septic tanks, sewage; erosion of natural deposits	10
IOC	Nitrite (measured as Nitrogen)	1	Infants below the age of six months who drink water containing nitrite in excess of the MCL could become seriously ill and, if untreated, may die Symptoms include shortness of breath and blue-baby syndrome	Runoff from fertilizer use; leaching from septic tanks, sewage; erosion of natural deposits	1
OC	Oxamyl (Vydate)	0 2	Slight nervous system effects	Runoff/leaching from insecticide used on apples, potatoes, and tomatoes	0 2
OC	Pentachlorophenol	0 001	Liver or kidney problems; increased cancer risk	Discharge from wood-preserving factories	zero
OC	Picloram	0 5	Liver problems	Herbicide runoff	0 5
OC	Polychlorinated biphenyls (PCBs)	0 0005	Skin changes; thymus gland problems; immune deficiencies reproductive or nervous system difficulties increased risk of cancer	Runoff from landfills discharge of waste chemicals	zero
R	Radium 226 and Radium 228 (combined)	5 pCi/L	Increased risk of cancer	Erosion of natural deposits	zero
IOC	Selenium	0 05	Hair or fingernai loss; numbness in fingers or toes; circulatory problems	Discharge from petroleum and metal refineries; erosion of natural deposits; discharge from mines	0 05
OC	Simazine	0 004	Problems with blood	Herbicide runoff	0 004
OC	Styrene	0 1	Liver, kidney, or circulatory system problems	Discharge from rubber and plastic factories; leaching from landfill	0 1
OC	Tetrachloroethylene	0 005	Liver problems; increased risk of cancer	Discharge from factories and dry cleaners	zero
IOC	Thallium	0 002	Hair loss; changes in blood; kidney, intestine, or liver problems	Leaching from ore-processing sites; discharge from electronics, glass, and drug factories	0 0005
OC	Toluene	1	Nervous system, kidney, or liver problems	Discharge from petroleum factories	1
M	Total Coliforms	5 0 percent[8]	Coliforms are bacteria that indicate that other, potentially harmful bacteria may be present See fecal coliforms and *E. coli*	Naturally present in the environment	zero
DBP	Total Trihalomethanes (TTHMs)	0 080	Liver, kidney or central nervous system problems; increased risk of cancer	Byproduct of drinking water disinfection	n/a[9]
OC	Toxaphene	0 003	Kidney, liver, or thyroid problems; increased risk of cancer	Runoff/leaching from insecticide used on cotton and cattle	zero
OC	2,4,5-TP (Silvex)	0 05	Liver problems	Residue of banned herbicide	0 05
OC	1,2,4-Trichlorobenzene	0 07	Changes in adrenal glands	Discharge from textile finishing factories	0 07
OC	1,1,1-Trichloroethane	0 2	Liver, nervous system, or circulatory problems	Discharge from metal degreasing sites and other factories	0 2
OC	1,1,2-Trichloroethane	0 005	Liver, kidney, or immune system problems	Discharge from industrial chemical factories	0 003
OC	Trichloroethylene	0 005	Liver problems; increased risk of cancer	Discharge from metal degreasing sites and other factories	zero

25

LEGEND

D Disinfectant	**IOC** Inorganic Chemical	**OC** Organic Chemical	
DBP Disinfection Byproduct	**M** Microorganism	**R** Radionuclides	

Safe Drinking Water Hotline: 800-426-4791

Contaminant		MCL or TT[1] (mg/L)[2]	Potential health effects from long-term[3] exposure above the MCL	Common sources of contaminant in drinking water	Public Health Goal (mg/L)[2]
M	Turbidity	TT[7]	Turbidity is a measure of the cloudiness of water It is used to indicate water quality and filtratio effectiveness (e g , whether disease-causing organisms are present) Higher turbidity levels are often associated with higher levels of disease-causing microorganisms such as viruses, parasites and some bacteria These organisms can cause short term symptoms such as nausea, cramps, diarrhea, and associated headaches	Soil runoff	n/a
R	Uranium	30µg/L	Increased risk of cancer, kidney toxicity	Erosion of natural deposits	zero
OC	Vinyl chloride	0 002	Increased risk of cancer	Leaching from PVC pipes; discharge from plastic factories	zero
M	Viruses (enteric)	TT[7]	Short-term exposure: Gastrointestinal illness (e g , diarrhea, vomiting, cramps)	Human and animal fecal waste	zero
OC	Xylenes (total)	10	Nervous system damage	Discharge from petroleum factories; discharge from chemical factories	10

26

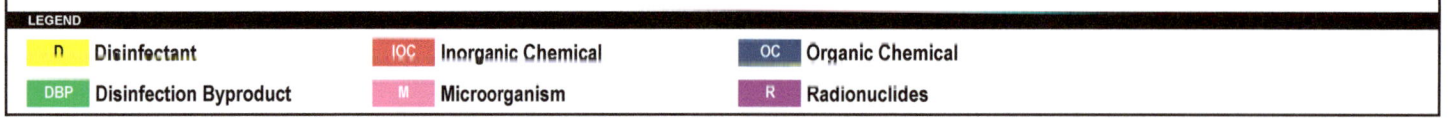

LEGEND

D Disinfectant	IOC Inorganic Chemical	OC Organic Chemical
DBP Disinfection Byproduct	M Microorganism	R Radionuclides

NOTES

1 Definitions

- Maximum Contaminant Level Goal (MCLG)—The level of a contaminant in drinking water below which there is no known or expected risk to health. MCLGs allow for a margin of safety and are non-enforceable public health goals.
- Maximum Contaminant Level (MCL)—The highest level of a contaminant that is allowed in drinking water. MCLs are set as close to MCLGs as feasible using the best available treatment technology and taking cost into consideration. MCLs are enforceable standards.
- Maximum Residual Disinfectant Level Goal (MRDLG)—The level of a drinking water disinfectant below which there is no known or expected risk to health. MRDLGs do not reflect the benefits of the use of disinfectants to control microbial contaminants.
- Maximum Residual Disinfectant Level (MRDL)—The highest level of a disinfectant allowed in drinking water. There is convincing evidence that addition of a disinfectant is necessary for control of microbial contaminants.
- Treatment Technique (TT)—A required process intended to reduce the level of a contaminant in drinking water.

2 Units are in milligrams per liter (mg/L) unless otherwise noted. Milligrams per liter are equivalent to parts per million (ppm).

3 Health effects are from long-term exposure unless specified as short-term exposure.

4 Each water system must certify annually, in writing, to the state (using third-party or manufacturers certification) that when it uses acrylamide and/or epichlorohydrin to treat water, the combination (or product) of dose and monomer level does not exceed the levels specified, as follows: Acrylamide = 0.05 percent dosed at 1 mg/L (or equivalent); Epichlorohydrin = 0.01 percent dosed at 20 mg/L (or equivalent).

5 Lead and copper are regulated by a Treatment Technique that requires systems to control the corrosiveness of their water. If more than 10 percent of tap water samples exceed the action level, water systems must take additional steps. For copper, the action level is 1 3 mg/L, and for lead is 0 015 mg/L.

6 A routine sample that is fecal coliform-positive or *E. coli*-positive triggers repeat samples--if any repeat sample is total coliform-positive, the system has an acute MCL violation. A routine sample that is total coliform-positive and fecal coliform-negative or *E. coli*-negative triggers repeat samples--if any repeat sample is fecal coliform-positive or *E. coli*-positive, the system has an acute MCL violation. See also Total Coliforms.

7 EPA's surface water treatment rules require systems using surface water or ground water under the direct influence of surface water to (1) disinfect their water, and (2) filter their water or meet criteria for avoiding filtration so that the following contaminants are controlled at the following levels:

- *Cryptosporidium*: 99 percent removal for systems that filter. Unfiltered systems are required to include Cryptosporidium in their existing watershed control provisions.
- Giardia lamblia: 99 9 percent removal/inactivation

- Viruses: 99.99 percent removal/inactivation
- *Legionella*: No limit, but EPA believes that if *Giardia* and viruses are removed/inactivated according to the treatment techniques in the surface water treatment rule, *Legionella* will also be controlled.
- Turbidity: For systems that use conventional or direct filtration, at no time can turbidity (cloudiness of water) go higher than 1 nephelolometric turbidity unit (NTU), and samples for turbidity must be less than or equal to 0.3 NTU in at least 95 percent of the samples in any month. Systems that use filtration other than conventional or direct filtration must follow state limits, which must include turbidity at no time exceeding 5 NTU.
- HPC: No more than 500 bacterial colonies per milliliter
- Long Term 1 Enhanced Surface Water Treatment; Surface water systems or ground water systems under the direct influence of surface water serving fewer than 10,000 people must comply with the applicable Long Term 1 Enhanced Surface Water Treatment Rule provisions (e g. turbidity standards, individual filter monitoring, *Cryptosporidium* removal requirements, updated watershed control requirements for unfiltered systems).
- Long Term 2 Enhanced Surface Water Treatment; This rule applies to all surface water systems or ground water systems under the direct influence of surface water. The rule targets additional *Cryptosporidium* treatment requirements for higher risk systems and includes provisions to reduce risks from uncovered finished water storages facilities and to ensure that the systems maintain microbial protection as they take steps to reduce the formation of disinfection byproducts. (Monitoring start dates are staggered by system size. The largest systems (serving at least 100,000 people) will begin monitoring in October 2006 and the smallest systems (serving fewer than 10,000 people) will not begin monitoring until October 2008. After completing monitoring and determining their treatment bin, systems generally have three years to comply with any additional treatment requirements.)
- Filter Backwash Recycling: The Filter Backwash Recycling Rule requires systems that recycle to return specific recycle flows through all processes of the system's existing conventional or direct filtration system or at an alternate location approved by the state.

8 No more than 5.0 percent samples total coliform-positive in a month. (For water systems that collect fewer than 40 routine samples per month, no more than one sample can be total coliform-positive per month.) Every sample that has total coliform must be analyzed for either fecal coliforms or *E. coli*. If two consecutive TC-positive samples, and one is also positive for *E. coli* or fecal coliforms, system has an acute MCL violation.

9 Although there is no collective MCLG for this contaminant group, there are individual MCLGs for some of the individual contaminants:

- Haloacetic acids: dichloroacetic acid (zero); trichloroacetic acid (0.3 mg/L)
- Trihalomethanes: bromodichloromethane (zero); bromoform (zero); dibromochloromethane (0.06 mg/L)

Appendix B: References

US EPA Publications

25 Years of the Safe Drinking Water Act: History & Trends
EPA 816-R-99-007

Community Water Systems Survey 2000, Volume I
EPA 815-R-02-0054

Drinking Water Costs and Federal Funding
EPA 810-F-99-014

Drinking Water from Household Wells
EPA 816-K-02-003

Drinking Water Priority Rulemaking: Microbial and Disinfection Byproduct Rules
EPA 816-F-01-012

Drinking Water Treatment
EPA 810-F-99-013

Factoids: Drinking Water and Ground Water Statistics for 2001
EPA 815-K-02-004

Factoids: Drinking Water and Ground Water Statistics for 2002
EPA 816–K-03-001

Fact Sheet: 1999 Drinking Water Infrastructure Needs Survey
EPA 816-F-01-001

"Investing in America's Water Infrastructure" Keynote Address by G. Tracy Mehan III to the Schwab Capital Markets' Global Water Conference
Protect Your Drinking Water
EPA 816-F-02-012

Public Access to Information & Public Involvement
EPA 810-F-99-021

Report to Congress: EPA Studies on Sensitive Subpopulations and Drinking Water Contaminants
EPA 815-R-00-015
Safe Drinking Water Act-Protecting America's Public Health
EPA 816-H-02-003

Safe Drinking Water Act: Underground Injection Control Program: Protecting Public Health and Drinking Water Resources
EPA 816-H-01-003

The Clean Water and Drinking Water Infrastructure Gap Analysis
EPA 816-F-02-017

The Drinking Water State Revolving Fund: Protecting the Public Through Drinking Water Infrastructure Improvements
EPA 819-F-00-028

Understanding the Safe Drinking Water Act
EPA 810-F-99-008

Using Water Wisely in the Home
EPA 800-F-02-001

Featured Consumer Information Resources

Download the following documents from EPA's New Drinking Water Consumer Information Web site: http://www.epa.gov/safewater/con-sumerinformation/

Or order hard copies from EPA's National Service Center for Environmental Publications:
 HYPERLINK "http://www.epa.gov/nscep" http://www.epa.gov/nscep or 1-800-490-9198

Public Health and Emergency Information:

Bottled Water Basics, 816-K-05-003

Filtration Facts, 816-K-05-002

Emergency Disinfection of Drinking Water
English, 816-F-06-027
Spanish, EPA 816-F-06-028
French, 816-F-06-045
Arabic, 816-F-06-030
Vietnamese, 816-F-06-029

What to Do After the Flood
English, 816-F-05-021
Spanish, 816-F-05-021
Vietnamese, 816-F-05-025

Is There Lead In My Drinking Water?
816-F-05-001

Guidance for People with Severely Weakened Immune Systems, 816-F-99-005

Public Involvement in Water Security Web site, a compilation of resources to help increase public awareness of water security issues and to give citizens information and guidance to help them prepare for potential emergency incidents and incorporate security activities into their daily lives, http://cfpub.epa.gov/safewater/water-security/publicInvolve.cfm

Environmental Education:

Thirstin's Drinking Water Games and Activities (CD-ROM), 816-C-04-008

Virtual Tour of a Water Treatment Plant (CD-ROM), 816-C-06-002

Find answers to your questions about drinking water and ground water programs authorized under the Safe Drinking Water Act in EPA's dynamic question and answer database, http://www.epa.gov/safewater/drin-klink.html.

Publications From Outside Sources

Centers for Disease Control and Prevention. Morbidity and Mortality Weekly Report: Surveillance for Waterborne-Disease Outbreaks-United States-1999-2000.

Congressional Budget Office. Future Investment in Drinking Water & Wastewater Infrastructure

Appendix D: Glossary

Action Level

The level of lead and copper which, if exceeded, triggers treatment or other requirements that a water system must follow.

Aquifer

A natural underground layer, often of sand or gravel, that contains water

Coliform

A group of related bacteria whose presence in drinking water may indicate contamination by disease-causing microorganisms

Community Water System (CWS)

A water system that supplies drinking water to 25 people or more year-round in their residences

Contaminant

Anything found in water (including microorganisms, radionuclides, chemicals, minerals, etc.) which may be harmful to human health

Cryptosporidium

Microorganism found commonly in lakes and rivers which is highly resistant to disinfection.

Disinfectant

A chemical (commonly chlorine, chloramines, or ozone) or physical process (e.g., ultraviolet light) that kills microorganisms such as viruses, bacteria, and protozoa

Distribution System

A network of pipes leading from a treatment plant to customers' plumbing systems

Ground Water

Water that is pumped and treated from an aquifer

Inorganic Contaminants

Mineral-based compounds such as metals, nitrates, and asbestos; naturally occurring in some water, but can also enter water through human activities

Maximum Contaminant Level

The highest level of a contaminant that EPA allows in drinking water (legally enforceable standard)

Maximum Contaminant Level Goal

The level of a contaminant at which there would be no risk to human health (not a legally enforceable standard)

Microorganisms

Tiny living organisms that can be seen only under a microscope; some can cause acute health problems when consumed in drinking water

Non-Transient Non-Community Water System

A non-community water system that serves the same people more than six months of the year, but not year-round

Organic Contaminants

Carbon-based chemicals, such as solvents and pesticides, which enter water through cropland runoff or discharge from factories

Pathogen

Disease-causing organism

Public Water System (PWS)

A water system which supplies drinking water to at least 25 people, at least 60 days each year

Sensitive Subpopulation

People who may be more vulnerable to drinking water contamination, such as infants, children, some elderly, and people with severely compromised immune systems

Septic System

Used to treat sanitary waste; can be a significant threat to water quality due to leaks or runoff

Source Water

Water in its natural state, prior to any treatment for drinking (i.e., lakes, streams, ground water)

Surface Water

Water that is pumped and treated from sources open to the atmosphere, such as rivers, lakes, and reservoirs

Transient Non-Community Water System

A non-community water system that serves the public but not the same individuals for more than six months

Violation

Failure to meet any state or federal drinking water regulation

Vulnerability Assessment

An evaluation of drinking water source quality and its vulnerability to contamination by pathogens and toxic chemicals

Watershed

The land area from which water drains into a stream, river, or reservoir

Well

A bored, drilled or driven shaft whose depth is greater than the largest surface dimension, a dug hole whose depth is greater than the largest surface dimension, an improved sinkhole, or a subsurface fluid distribution system